A gift for you from...

_____

Facing Death

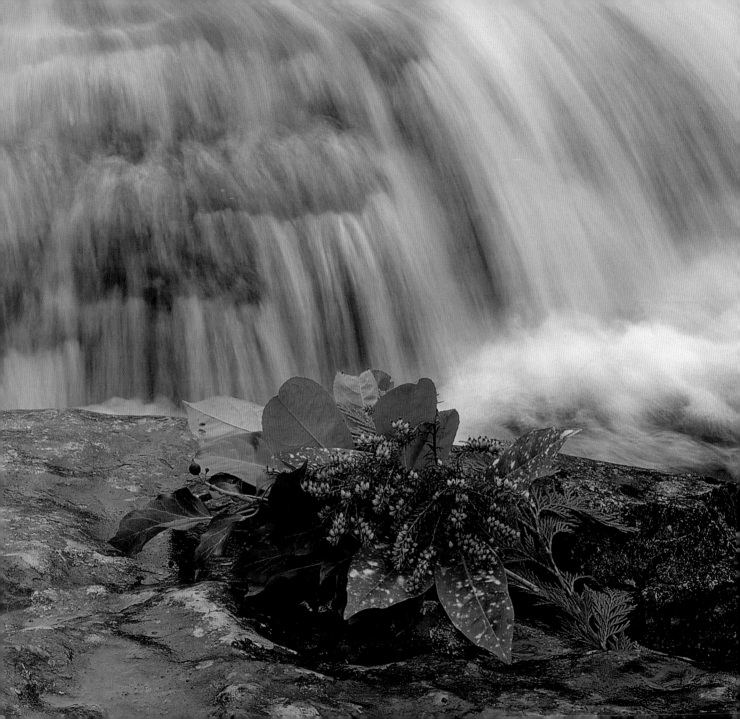

Facing Death

A COMPANION IN WORDS AND IMAGES

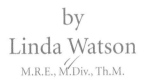

by

Linda Watson

M.R.E., M.Div., Th.M.

Photography by Maggie Sale

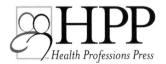
Health Professions Press

Baltimore • London • Sydney

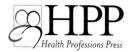

Health Professions Press, Inc.
Post Office Box 10624
Baltimore, Maryland 21285-0624

www.healthpropress.com

Interior and cover design by Joyce Weston Design.
Typeset by Joyce Weston.
Manufactured in China by Jade Productions.

Special arrangements are available for quantity purchases.
Contact Special Sales Department (rights@healthpropress.com
or 1-888-337-8808) for more information.

Library of Congress Cataloging-in-Publication Data
Watson, Linda, M.R.E.
    Facing death : a companion in words and images / by Linda
Watson ; photography by Maggie Sale.
        p. cm.
    Includes bibliographical references.
    ISBN 978-1-932529-48-7 (pbk.)
    1. Death. 2. Terminal care. 3. Death—Quotations, maxims,
etc. 4. Bereavement. I. Sale, Maggie. II. Title.
    R726.8.W38 2009
    616′.029—dc22   2008054467

Contents

Dedicated to the memory of

Dorothy Heather-Mae Yates

1940–2003

Forever loved

Preface

*A*S WITH MANY THINGS IN LIFE, there is a story behind
this book. The year before I was diagnosed with cancer, my
eldest sister, Dorothy, was likewise diagnosed. Unfortunately, in her
case the cancer spread to various parts of her body within a few years.
One spring she was given six weeks to live.

I lived a distance away and was facing my own health challenges,
and so I could only rarely visit her. This was very frustrating to me,
especially because I knew that in addition to my great love for
Dorothy, I had skills, knowledge, and a degree of comfort in compan-
ioning the dying. I was, however, unable to share those with her fully.
I phoned regularly, but that was not enough.

It was out of this sense of frustration and a longing to make a difference that I conceived the idea of compiling favorite quotations,
scripture passages, and personal messages for Dorothy. I gave them to
her, asking simply that she at least read them through once and then
make use of them in whichever way felt appropriate to her.

To my surprise, Dorothy expressed to me a month later that she
was reading through the messages every day, as a kind of devotional
practice. They spoke to her. She found inspiration and comfort in
them. I was so pleased to know that they were making some of the
difference I had intended.

I was with Dorothy in her palliative care room in the last week of
her life, and at least once a day she asked me to read through the

messages I had collected for her. By then, some of the messages no longer seemed to speak to her situation, so we skipped those and focused on the remainder. My sister lived past the six weeks the doctors had predicted for her. In fact, she lived through five more months. I last read to her, at her request and with tears running down my face, one afternoon in late November. She died early the next morning.

I originally had no idea of sharing these messages with others. However, when I shared the concept with care professionals, I was encouraged to refine the messages for other people to use in facing the ultimate transition we call *death*.

Thus it is that you are holding this book in your hands today. If you are facing your own imminent death, then my wish for you, as it was for my sister, is this:

> *May you find comfort and inspiration.*
> *May you find the support you need.*
> *May you move toward acceptance,*
> *and may you find peace at the last.*

— Linda Watson

Introduction

*I*N POPULAR USAGE, the terms *living* and *dying* are considered polar opposites, the one exclusive of the other.

However, if you are one among those who has, because of advancing age or disease, come to a place of facing the reality of your own mortality, then you may know that the the two are not always mutually exclusive. You, or someone you love, may be living *now* with the awareness that death is not far off in the remote future, that it does in fact invade the present. In this way, dying and living accompany one another as part of the experience of the living.

This book is intended as a resource for you to use in ways that make sense to you, as you contemplate the near possibility of your own death or that of a loved one.

The original compilation that I created consisted of words only— strong, precious, helpful words, but still words alone. As I reworked the material in preparation for publication, I realized that although the words could stand on their own, they would be greatly enriched by the accompaniment of photographic images.

With this in mind, I approached a long-time friend and award-winning nature photographer, Maggie Sale, to see if we might collaborate on this project. Maggie's agreement came swift and certain. She could see the possibilities. She would be delighted to have her images associated with such a project. Although I had anticipated the "value-added" possibilities of images accompanying the text, nothing prepared me for the sheer power and brilliance of Maggie's artistry joined with the messages.

Please feel free to make use of this book in any way that is helpful to you.

We have provided words and images for you to consider, pages for your own written messages, and even pages to hold a few cherished pictures or mementos of your own. Feel free to personalize this book for yourself with bookmarks, notations, and other additions.

Use it alongside other materials or on its own. Use it privately for your own emotional and spiritual nourishment. Share it with family and friends. Read it together with loved ones and allow the moment to open you all to a deeper sharing of the experience you face. Discuss or make notes about some of the messages or images and why they speak to you, or how some miss the mark for you and why.

Suggestions for caregivers and care professionals can be found in the two sections that follow.

However you use the book, make it your own, and may something of grace and peace blossom for you in the process.

For Caregivers and Loved Ones

*I*T IS A VERY COMMON EXPERIENCE to be at a loss for words in the presence of one who is facing the end of life. Sometimes, intensity of affection can make it harder rather than easier to talk about imminent passing, partly because we do not want to admit it is near.

We may feel in our hearts, however illogical it may seem, that talking about death will make it happen.

We may be reluctant to upset whatever delicate balance is helping the one for whom we care "keep it together" as the days and months pass.

We may be afraid that such talk will distress the very one we seek to support.

We may fear losing emotional control ourselves if we start talking about what is really happening.

We may be waiting for a signal from the one whose passing is drawing nearer every day.

Facing Death may help supply the words we are sometimes at a loss to find. Giving the book as a gift may say all that needs to be said. There are also ways you can personalize the book, if you desire.

You could add a personal note on the gift page at the front of the book.

You could insert quotations or personal messages on any of the photo-only pages at the end of Part One.

You could record your own thoughts and reflections on the lined pages in Part Two: My Reflections.

You could attach treasured pictures, notes, and other items of meaning to the blank pages provided in Part Three: My Pictures.

In addition, you could offer to read the messages aloud to your friend or loved one. If the situation seems right, you could ask what passages or pictures have the most appeal and why. You may find that such conversations lead to meaningful exchanges that might not otherwise have taken place.

I would also encourage *you* to seek support—professional, personal, and/or spiritual—as you walk through this process with the person for whom you care. It is not an easy journey. It is not a simple vigil. It is my hope that the messages in this book provide comfort and support to you as well.

A Word to Care Professionals

*T*HE CONTENT OF *Facing Death*, while meaningful and accessible, is not intended to replace other forms of care and support. It can, however, be there when you are not and complement other materials you might use with your patient, client, or congregant. It may even be that the book nourishes *your* spirit as you seek to be a helpful companion to the one in your care. You are encouraged to draw attention to particular parts of the book that the person in your care may need guidance in using.

The material encompasses at least three broad categories. First, it contains messages that are practical, even instructional, in nature. Second, it includes material that addresses and validates the range of feelings experienced by those facing their own mortality. Third, it provides inspirational passages that are intended to offer comfort, encouragement, and, yes, hope in the context of the end-of-life experience.

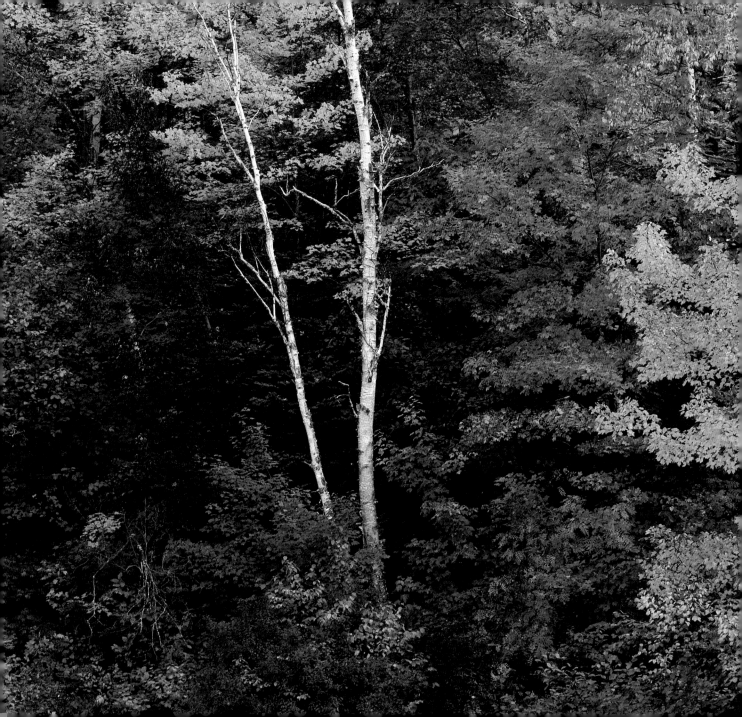

Part One

Thoughts and Images

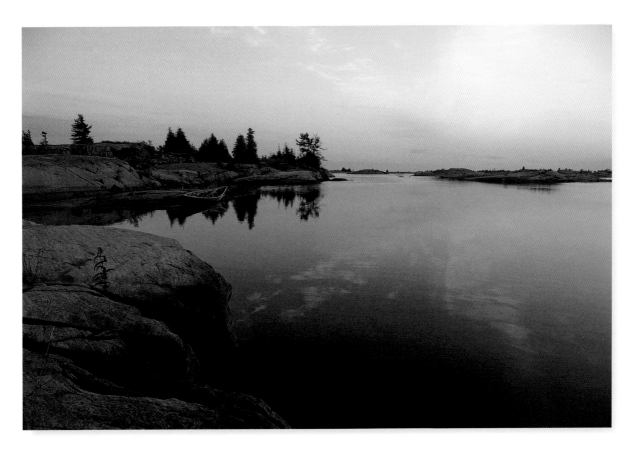

If you would die at peace,
then you must live at peace.
The good news is that it is not too late.
Reach out. Tell the truth. Forgive others.
Forgive yourself. Make amends.
Say the words "I love you."
Express gratitude.
Insofar as it lies within you,
make the peace you seek while you can.

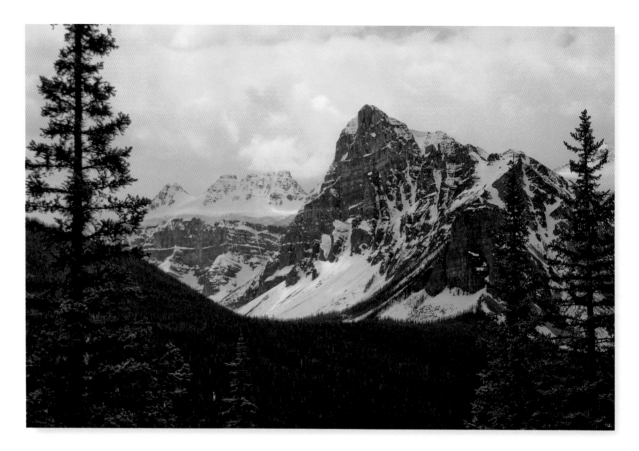

Of course,
you have every right to grieve.
After all, you are losing everything—
except, of course,
for who you are in yourself
and who you have been to others.
These things endure.

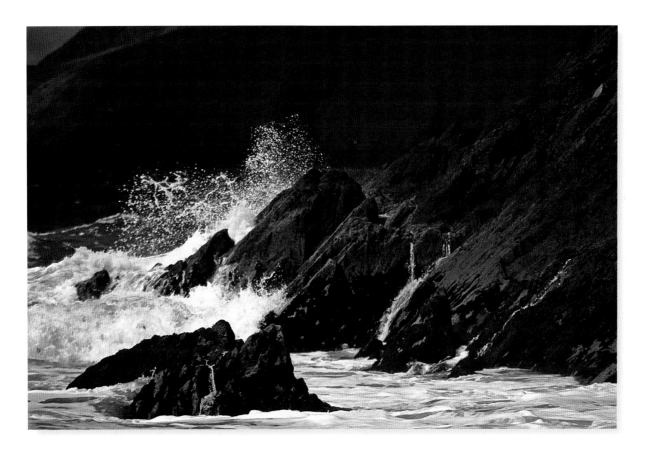

To weep, to rage,
to withdraw for a time—
these are demonstrations of grief.
They are not indications
of lack of faith or of a weak spirit.
These are proof of a living consciousness.
Grief is a holy thing
because it connects us to
that which is REAL.

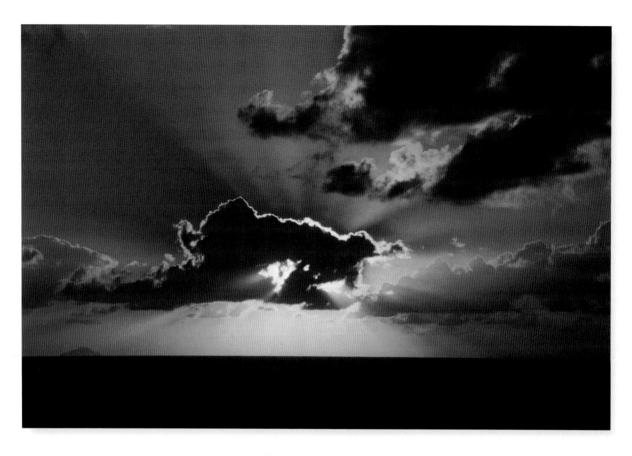

At death, if not before,
we get trimmed and pared,
and all that's left is the *loving*—
shining like an alive thing—
radiating into God.

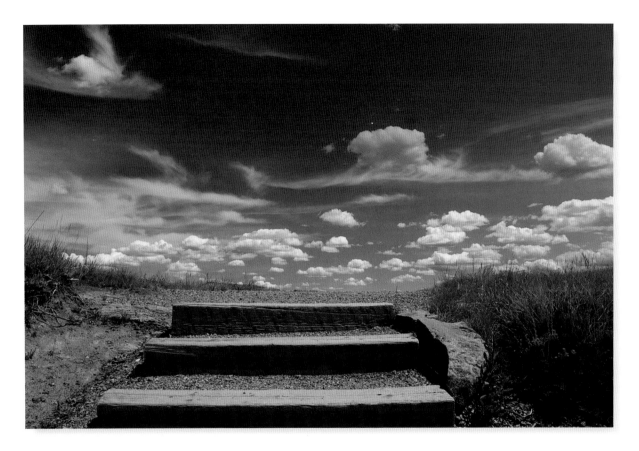

We are earth people
on a spiritual journey to the stars.
Our quest, our earth walk,
is to look within, to know who we are,
to see that we are connected to all things,
that there is no separation,
only in the mind.

—*Native American, source unknown*

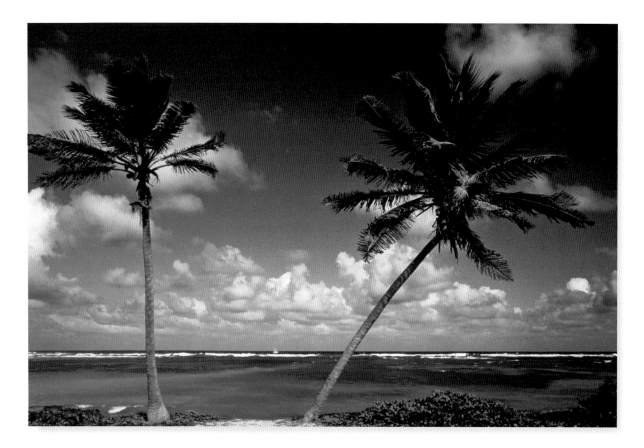

Healing is that which can make
the progress of disease,
even death itself,
approximately tolerable.
Healing is about spiritual wellness,
achieving inner peace,
and hope beyond sight.

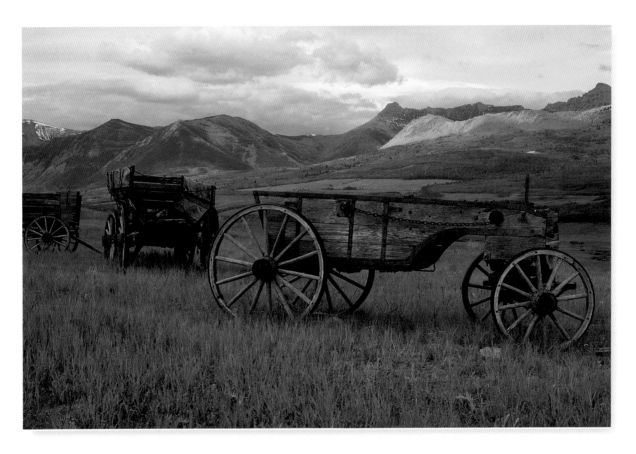

Many people
mistake courage for fearlessness.
Courage is the will to carry on and
the capacity to make the best
of the hand you have been dealt—
even when you are afraid.

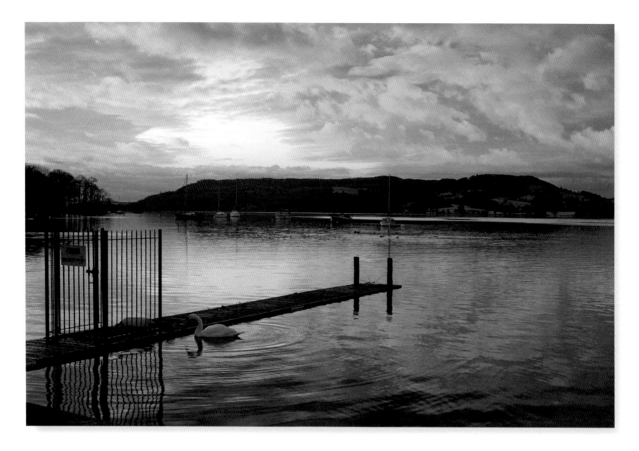

Use your time, now,
wisely and with clear intention.
Resolve relationships. Write letters.
Review your will.
Set down your preferences
for an observance of your passing.
This is a work of grieving
and of preparation.
It is also a Gift.

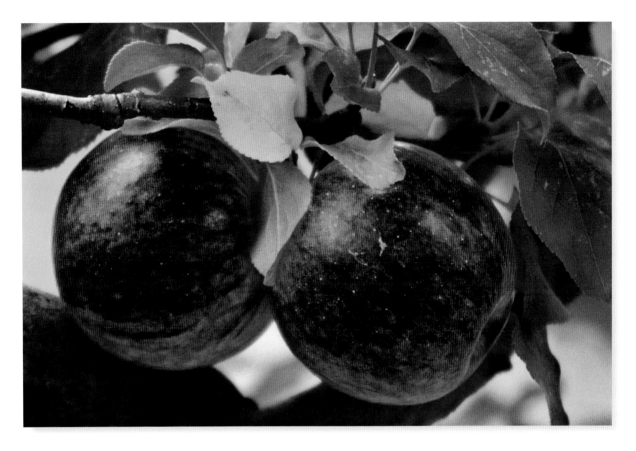

Life really is
a bittersweet confection,
is it not?
It can be bitter, confounding,
and filled with dread.
At the same time, it can be tantalizing,
delightful, and precious—
almost beyond belief.

You are loved.
You always will be loved.
It is a condition of your existence
in this universe.

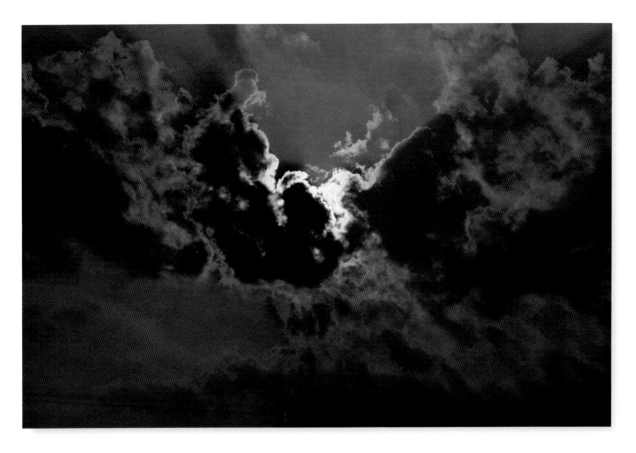

God, the Heart of the Universe,
that Higher Power, really is *here*—
right here and right now—
right here with you,
in the middle of this mess.

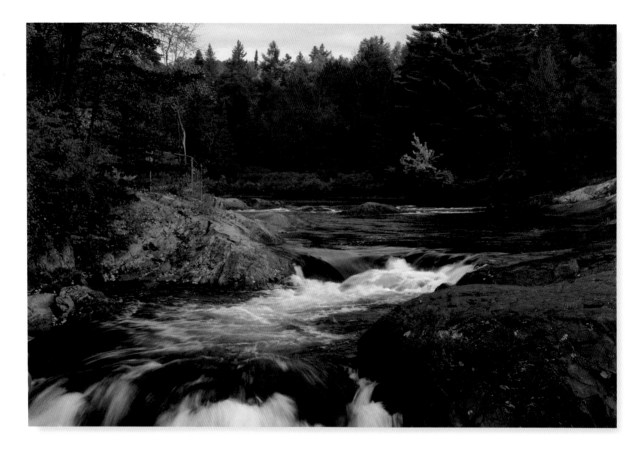

Do not fear, for I have redeemed you.
I called you by your name,
you are Mine.
When you pass through water,
I am with you,
and in rivers,
they shall not overflow you.

—*Jehovah, in the voice of the Prophet Isaiah*

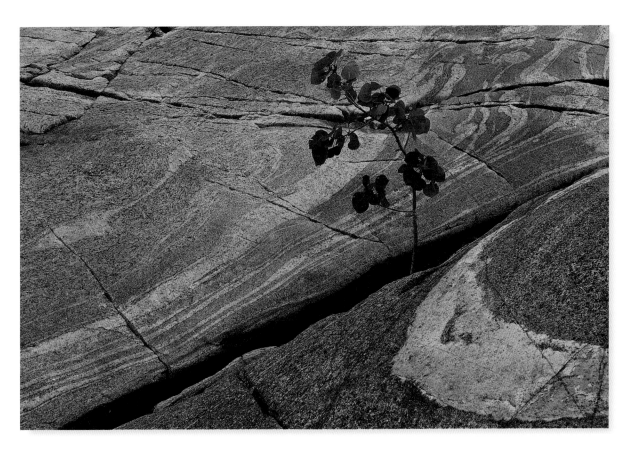

He did not say,
"You will not be troubled" or
"You will not have bitter labor" or
"You will have no discomfort," but
"You will not be overcome."

—*Julian of Norwich*

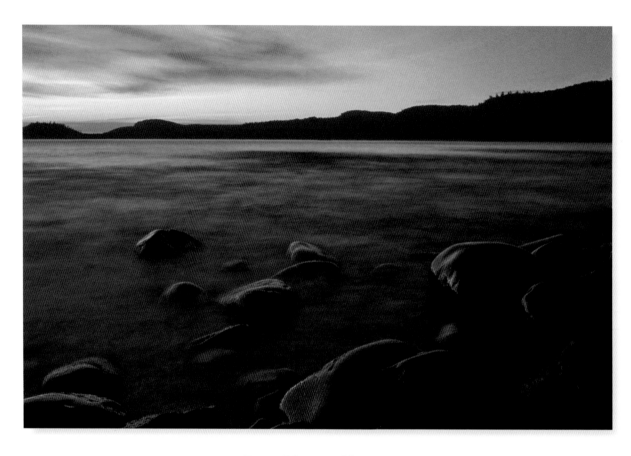

Peace I leave with you;
my peace I give to you.
I do not give to you as the world gives.
Do not let your hearts be troubled
and do not let them be afraid.

—Jesus

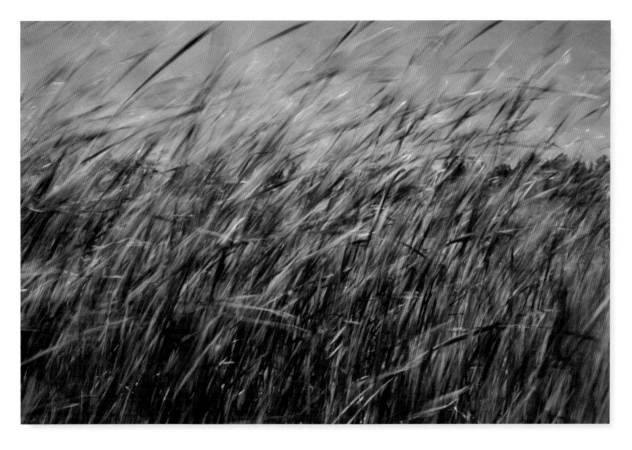

What is life?
It is the flash of a firefly in the night.
It is the breath of a buffalo
in the wintertime.
It is the little shadow
which runs across the grass and
loses itself in the sunset.

—*Crowfoot, Chief of the Blackfoot in the 1700s*

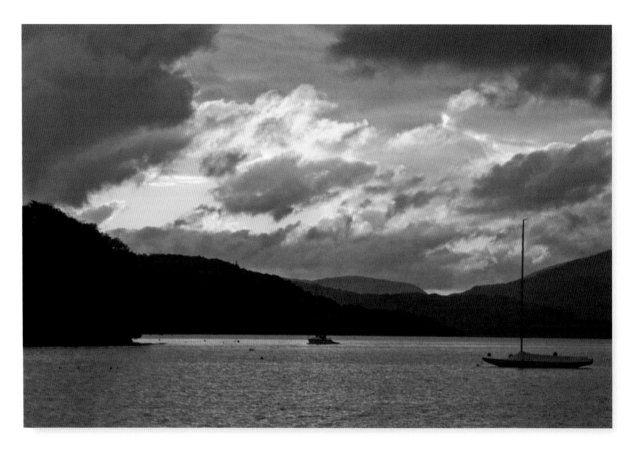

I have read about,
and I have personally known,
people who have experienced
"crossing over" to that Other Place.
Consistently, the report is
that what marks that crossing
is a sense of
all-encompassing welcome.

Express your grief.
Talk about it, cry it out,
pray it through.
You are entitled.

Dying at peace involves
the unlooked-for discovery that Death,
that long-despised Enemy,
can become, if not exactly a welcome friend,
at least a Deliverer
from the ongoing need to do battle.

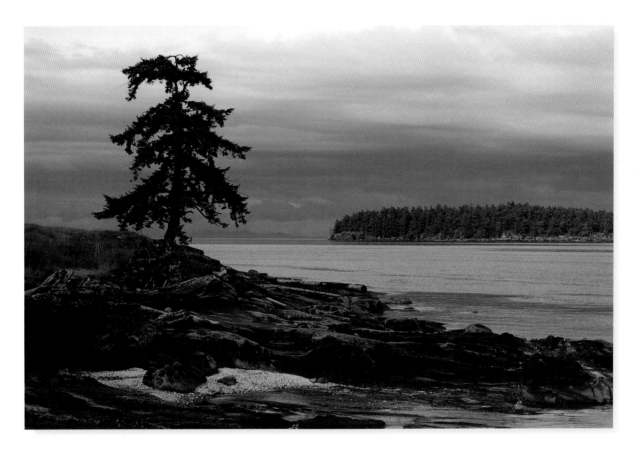

Of course,
good-byes become difficult,
even when you know
they are not yet final.
Every parting is a piercing reminder of
The Great Departing
awaiting you.
There is no relief from this.
It is part of the preparation.

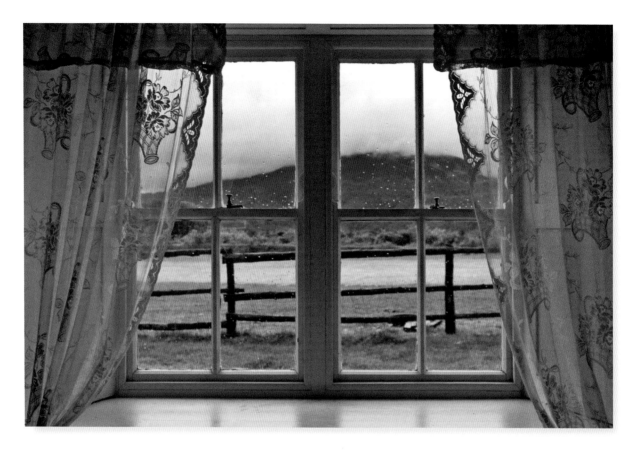

Dying at peace is possible.
All you need is time to prepare,
to let it sink in
and to say your "good-byes."
Dying at peace is possible and
some of its conditions are in your control.

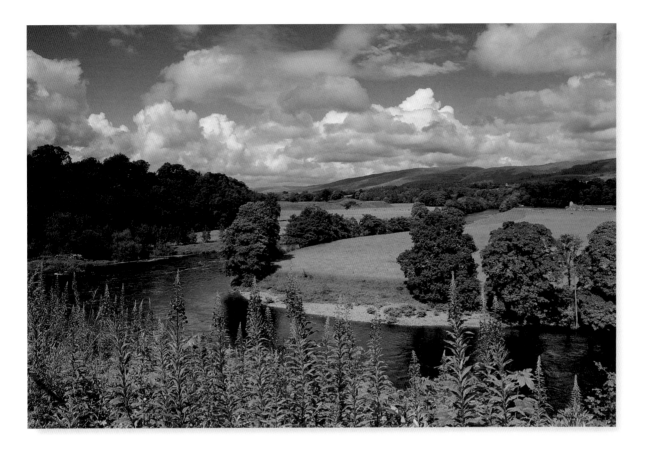

You have the dubious distinction of
knowing for certain
that your days are numbered.
Make every one of them count.
Greet each day with anticipation.
End each day with gratitude.
In between, do what you can.

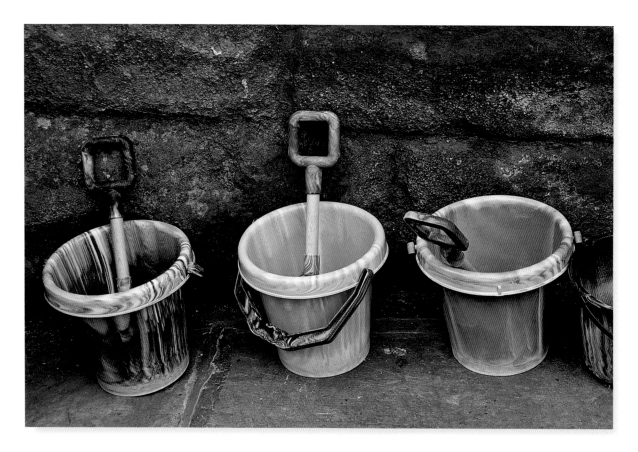

Use every precious moment
to create joyful, shared memories
with your friends and family.
Together you can fill a treasure chest
for all time.

—*Anne Knight*

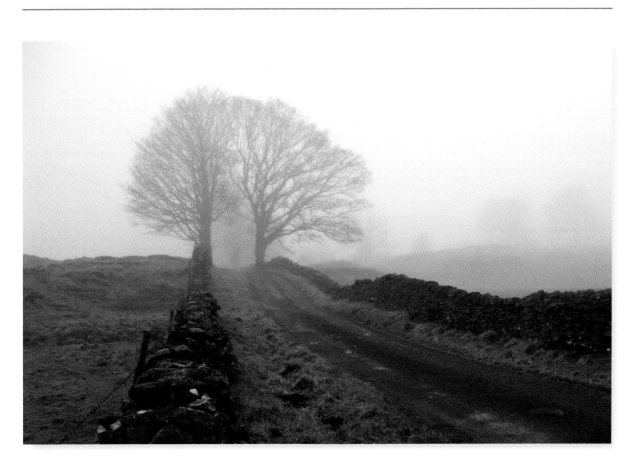

In some ways,
this journey you are on
must be the loneliest of all passages.
It is also an interlude
in which your oneness with all things
becomes exquisitely tangible.
Thus it is that, strangely,
when you feel most alone,
you are actually most companioned.

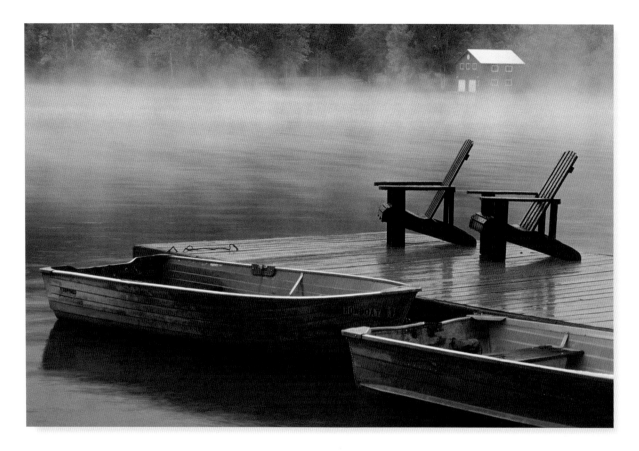

Pay attention.
Gather up moments of joy
and handle them again and again.
Tell stories. Laugh together.
Make memories.
Discover the holy in the day to day.

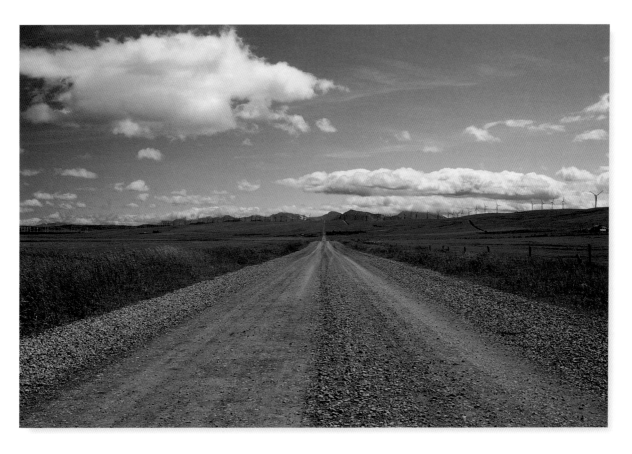

Life is eternal
and love is immortal;
and death is only a horizon,
and a horizon is nothing,
save the limit of our sight.

—*Rossiter Worthington Raymond*

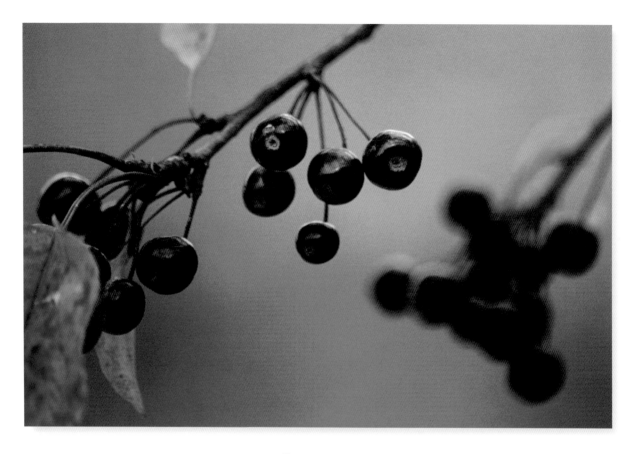

I *will* pay attention
to that which brings joy.
I *will* savor the beauty,
the tenderness, and
the happy surprises that come my way.
By these means, I *shall* Choose Life—
until the moment when that choice
means surrendering to death.

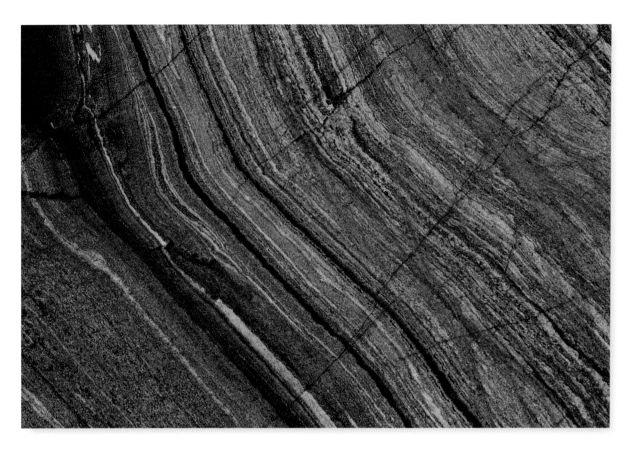

God does not cause our misfortunes.
Some are caused by bad luck,
some are caused by bad people,
and some are simply
an inevitable consequence
of our being human and being mortal,
living in a world of inflexible natural laws.

—*Rabbi Harold Kushner*

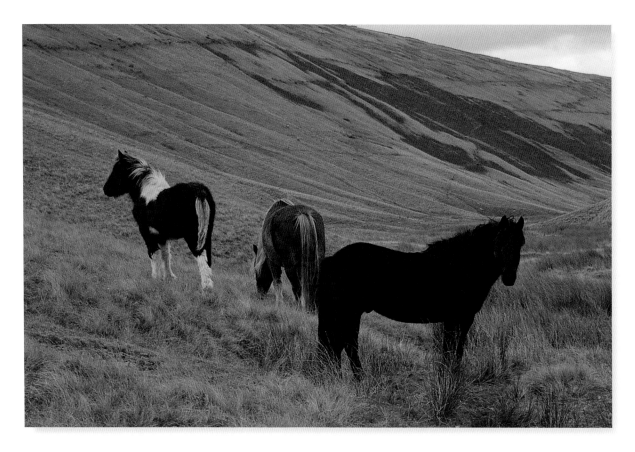

I put my trust in God,
My Lord and your Lord!
There is not a moving creature,
but He hath grasp of its forelock.

—*The Prophet Mohammed*

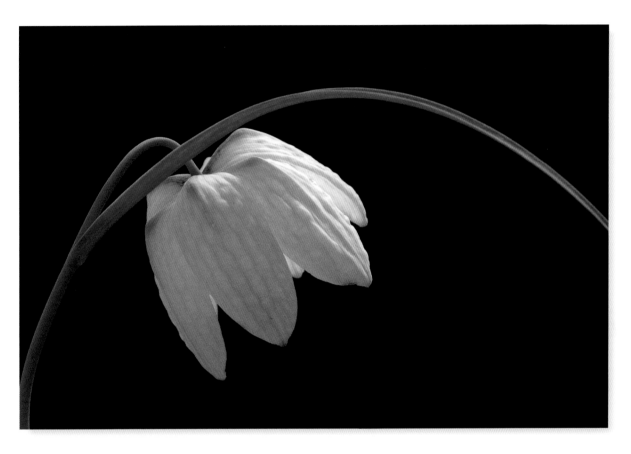

Choose your words well.
Express your feelings. Build others up.
You may be amazed at how others
will hang upon your words.
You would be even more amazed
if you could see what their impact will be
when you are gone.
Make them count for good.

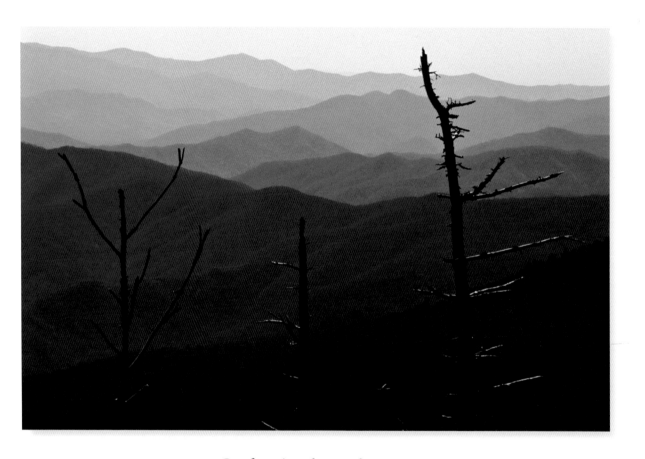

Confronting the randomness
that rules in this universe is painful.
Attempts to discover a
satisfyingly logical explanation
for what has happened to you—
up to and including blaming yourself—
is a reaction to this pain.

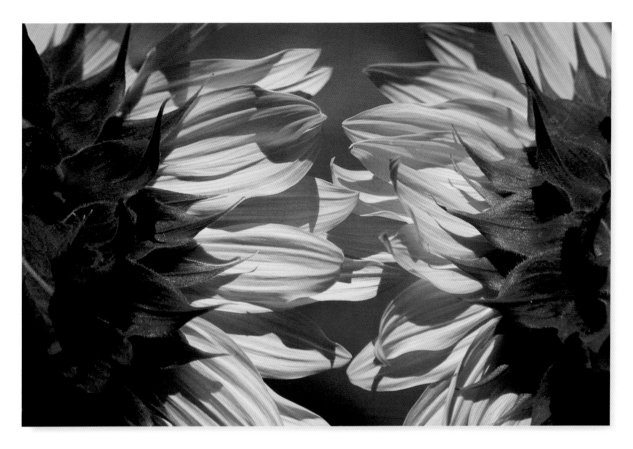

The specter of Death
is a great diviner of souls.
Some people will come across for you
in ways you might never have expected.
Latch onto these souls and
focus your energies with them.
Let the others
trickle through your fingers like sand
and entrust them to God.

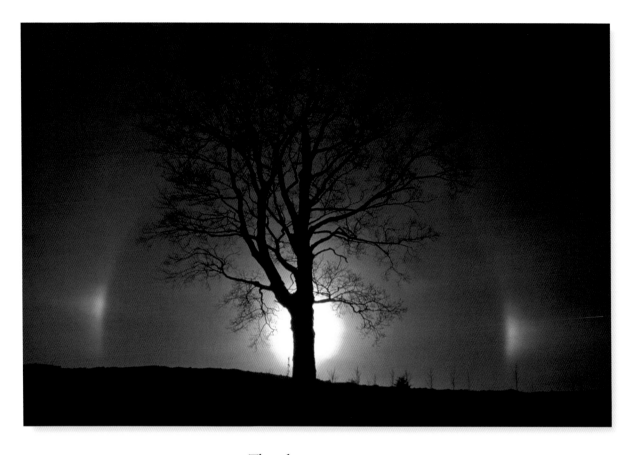

The place we are cast
when we face terror, dislocation,
life-threatening illness,
and the seeming absence of God,
has many names:
the Valley of the Shadow of Death,
the Void, the Pit of Despair, Hell itself.
It is also surely named Grief.

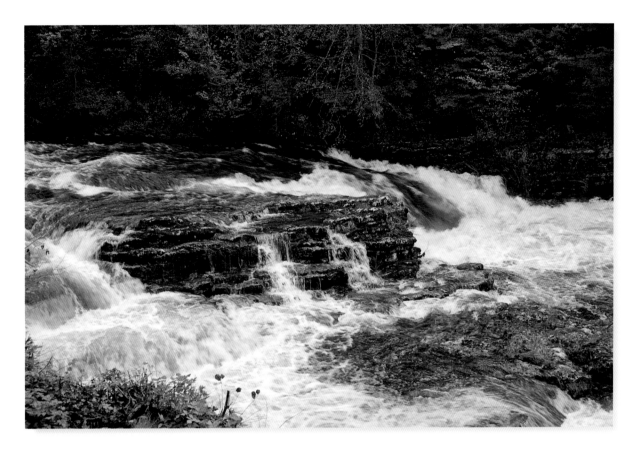

Freedom may come
not from being in control of life
but rather from a willingness
to move with the events of life,
to hold on to our memories
but let go of the past,
to choose, when necessary, the inevitable.
We can become free at any time.

—*Rachel Naomi Remen*

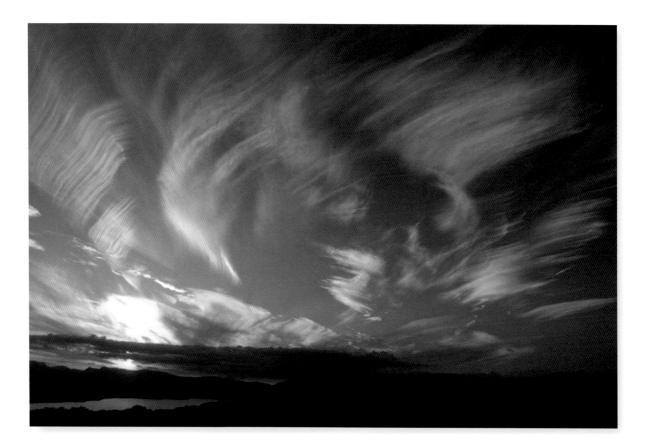

Where shall I go from Your spirit,
and where shall I flee from Your presence?
If I ascend to the heavens, there You are,
and if I make my bed in the grave, behold, You are there.
If I take up the wings of the dawn,
if I dwell at the end of the west,
there too, Your hand will lead me,
and Your right hand will grasp me.

—*The Psalmist*

Even when I walk in
the valley of darkness,
I will fear no evil
for You are with me;
Your rod and Your staff—
they comfort me.

—*The Psalmist*

I am convinced that neither death, nor life,
nor angels, nor rulers,
nor things present, nor things to come,
nor powers, nor height, nor depth,
nor anything else in all creation,
will be able to separate us
from the love of God
in Christ Jesus our Lord.

—*St. Paul*

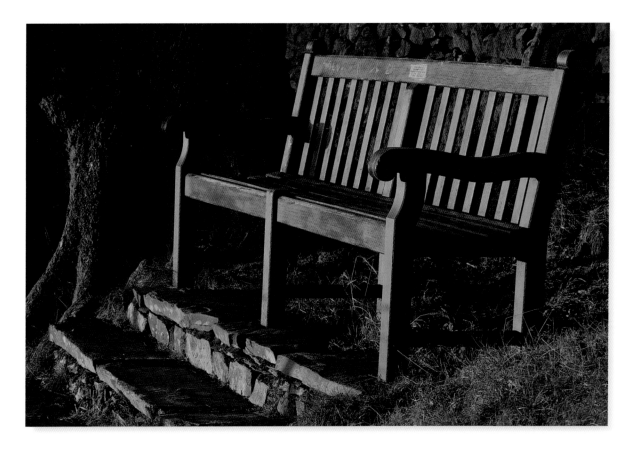

Death is not
extinguishing the light;
it is putting out the lamp
because dawn has come.

—Rabindranath Tagore, Bengali Poet

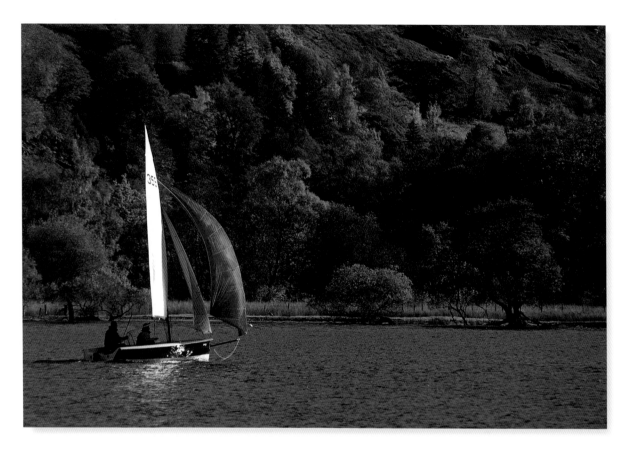

It's only when
we truly know and understand
that we have a limited time on earth—
and that we have no way of knowing
when our time is up—
that we will then begin
to live each day to the fullest,
as if it was the only one we had.

—*Elisabeth Kübler-Ross*

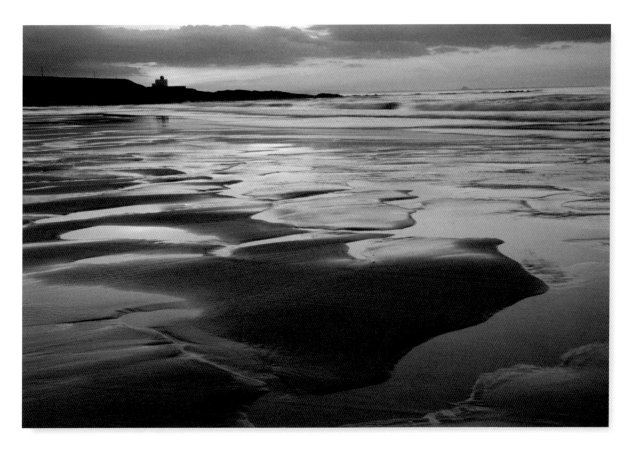

May you be blessed,
this day and every day,
with wisdom and understanding,
courage and commitment,
comfort and peace—
blessed by the Divine One
who has loved you into life
and who, even now,
lives you into hope.

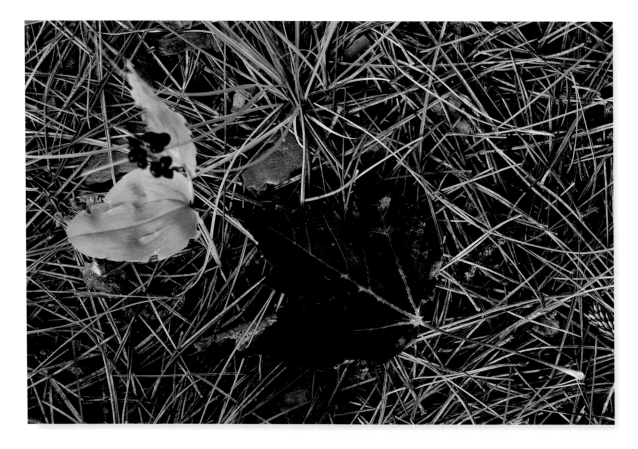

Paying attention—
to a leaf, a piece of music,
a sunset, a beloved face,
another's story, the unexpected,
an elder's hands, a child's questions—
is a sacred act.
For this we are made.

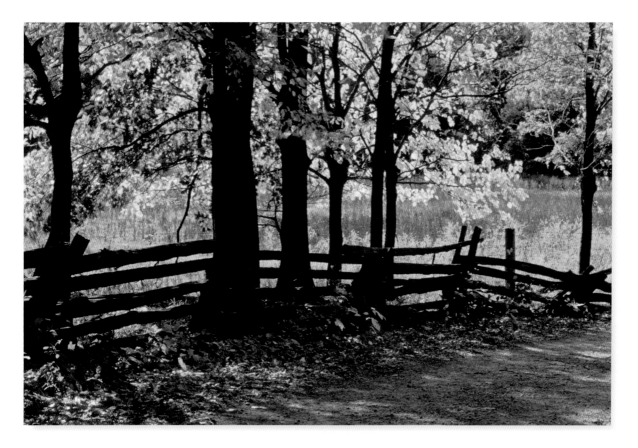

Along with relinquishing
precious freedoms,
a time will come when you have to let go
of any sense of responsibility you carry
for the choices, needs, and burdens of others.
That doesn't mean letting go of the relationships.
It just means trusting others
to attend to their own processes.

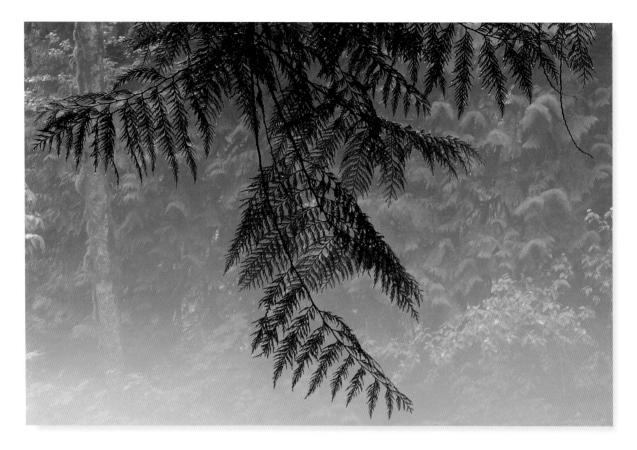

Teach me, Divine Presence,
that I may know—
taste, sense, understand,
and stand under—
hope,
in all its fragile beauty.

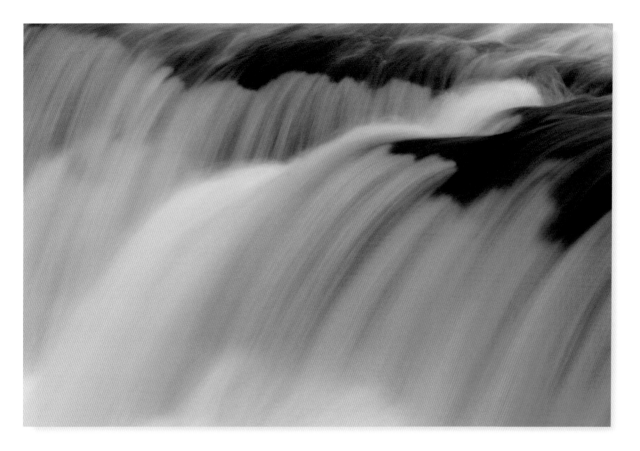

When you are angry, pound the pillows.
When you are sad, let the tears flow.
When you are frightened,
name your demons.
When you are anxious, make a list.
When you are alienated, seek support.
Honor your feelings.
They will guide you to
new discoveries and deeper peace.

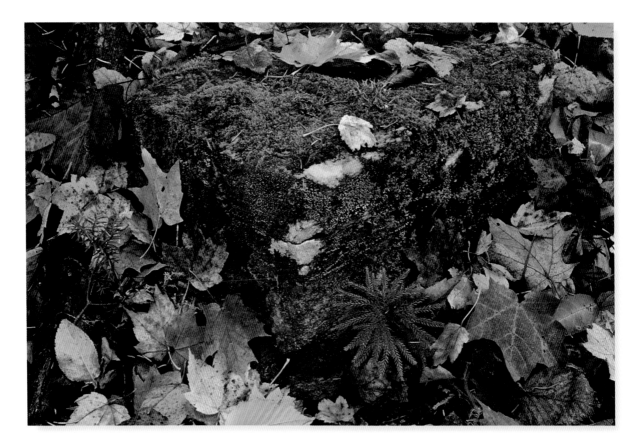

Few people today
know how to accompany the dying.
One of your tasks will be to set the tone
and to make your needs known.
Talk about it, for one thing.
It is probably safe to assume that others
are afraid to bring up the topic.
Accept offerings with grace.
You may be surprised by what greets you.

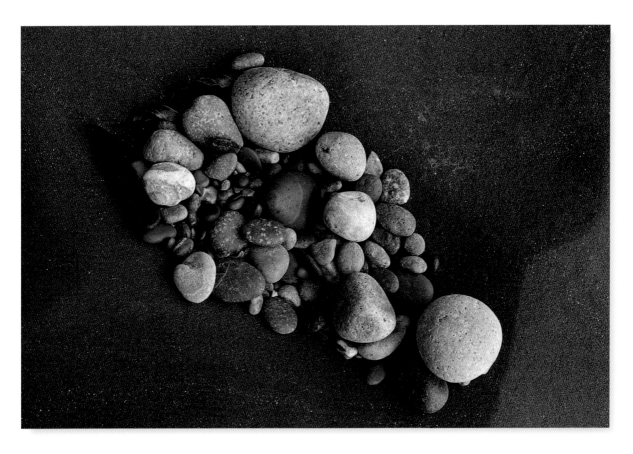

Age and disease
slowly erode the possibility of expressing
strength and independence fully,
as choices shift to other hands and
indignities overtake us.
Then we have opportunity
to acquire a new skill—namely,
the grace of receiving.

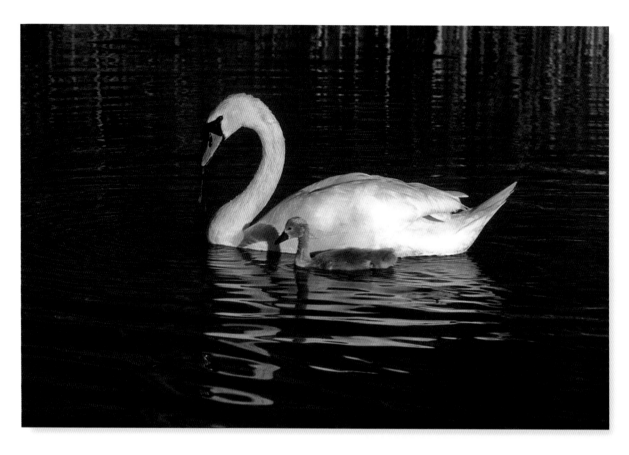

O, Divine Presence,
hold me to your breast.
Let me cling to you
and know the comfort
of your gentle love.
I am in need of tenderness.

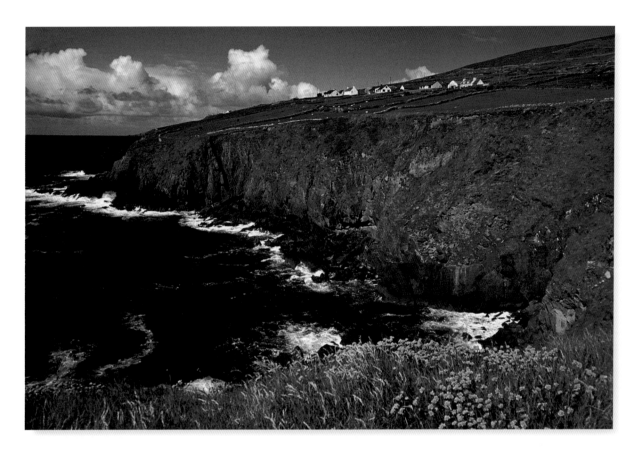

There is
an essential continuity
between this life and the next.
We prepare ourselves
for that latter mode of living
by making a practice of
living well
on this side of the divide.

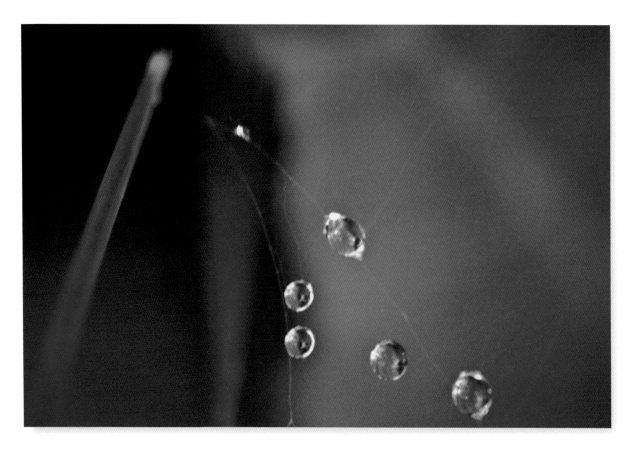

In my experience,
tears, fully and unselfconsciously shed,
are a powerful kind of prayer.
And, like all prayers,
they are the medium of surrender
to what some call God's will
and others call simply "what is."

—*Miriam Greenspan*

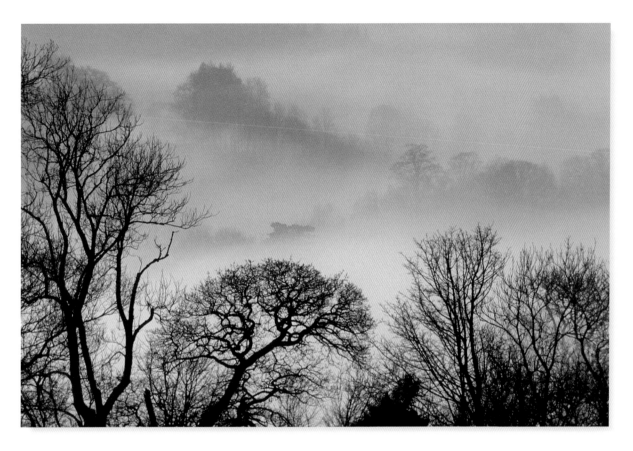

Likewise,
the Spirit helps us in our weakness;
for we do not know how
to pray as we ought,
but that very Spirit intercedes
with sighs too deep for words.

—St. Paul

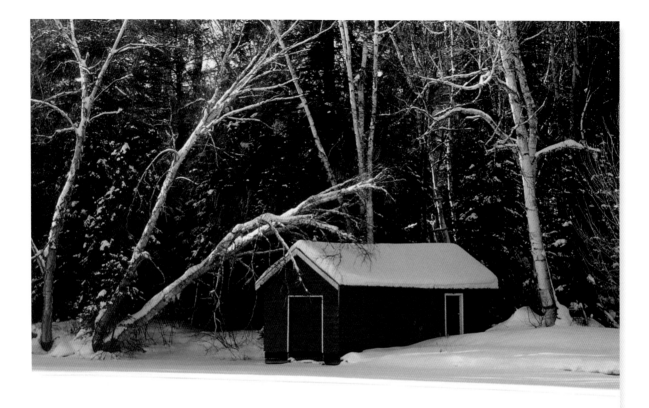

You do not have to go through this
alone.
In addition to friends and family,
there are spiritual support professionals
and communities you can turn to.
There are also "peer supports" available:
support groups, phone buddies.
Find the supports that suit you
and lean into them.

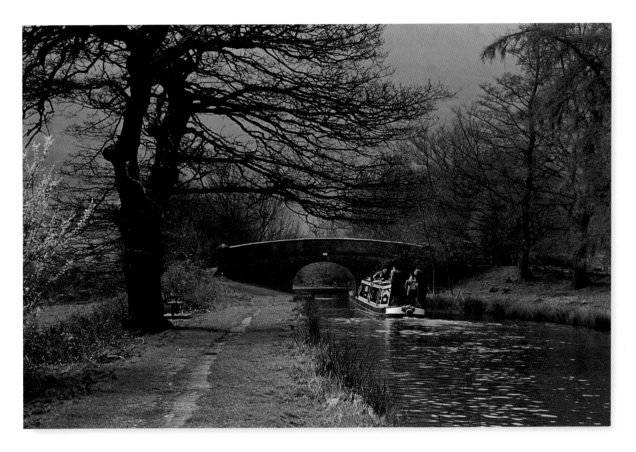

If you are faced with the choice
of whether or not to continue
active medical treatment,
don't let anyone assume the choice for you.
You have the right to persevere.
You have the right to call a halt.
It is your life.
Declare *your* wishes.

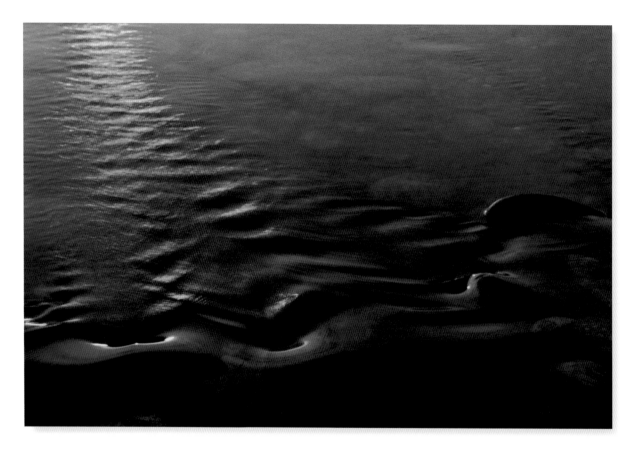

In large measure,
we are defined by our relationships.
If you have been given
some lead time on your dying,
attending to your relationships now
will bring peace and blessings
that trail after you
when you are gone.

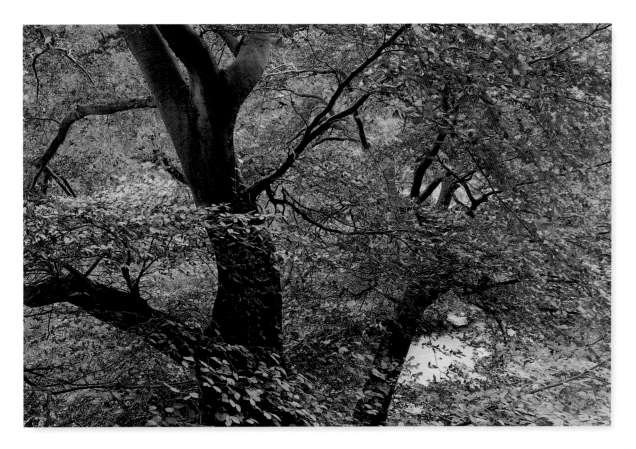

The real gift
of experiencing life-threatening illness
is that you have the opportunity
to confront your own mortality
in time.

—*Arlene Cotter*

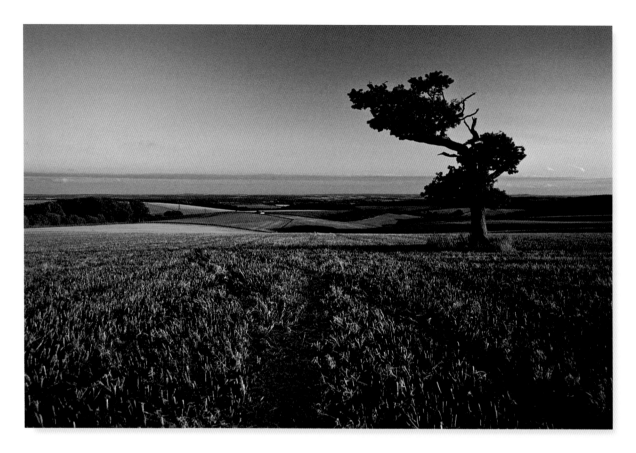

Love is the soul of life.
I, at least, am persuaded that,
even as the Life of the Spirit
does not end at the horizon
we call physical death,
so too, the Landscape of Love
broadens out forever.

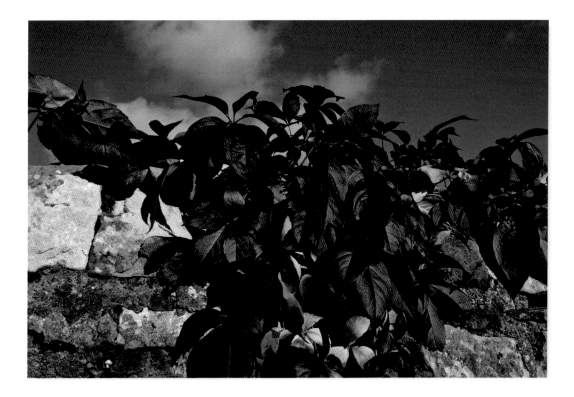

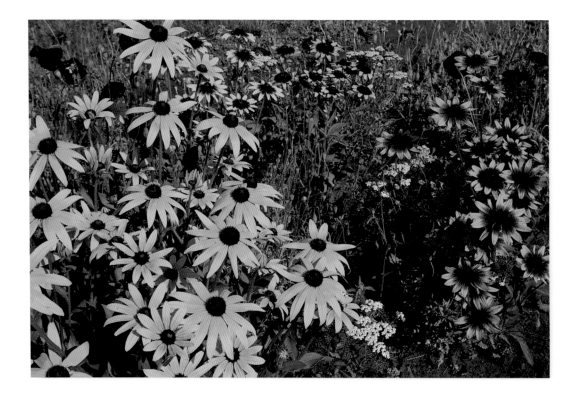

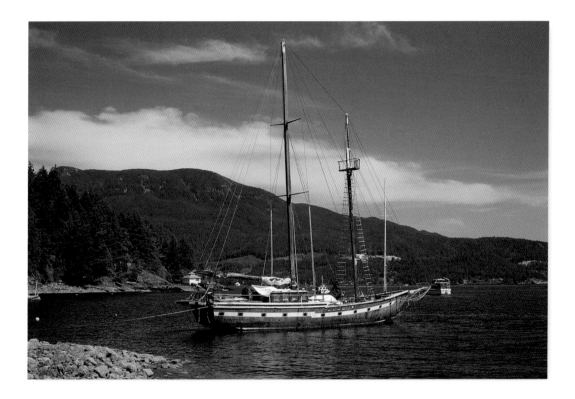

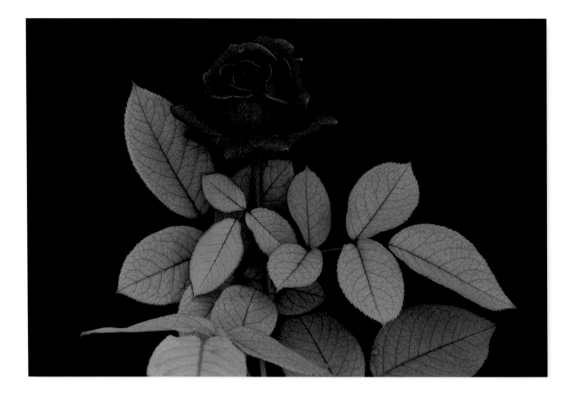

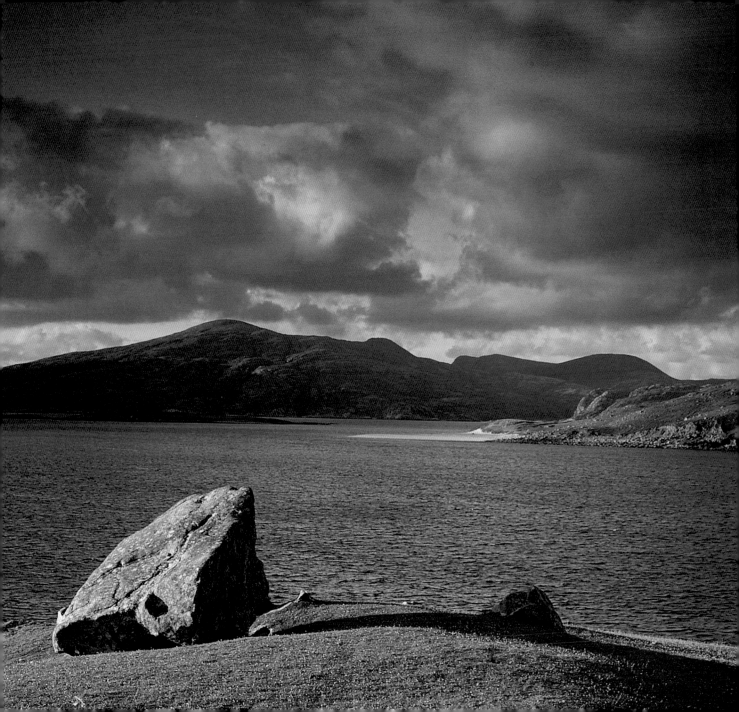

Part Two

My Reflections

Record your own thoughts
and reflections.

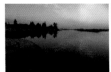

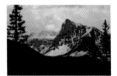

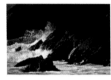

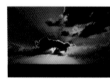

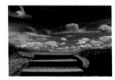

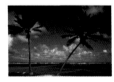

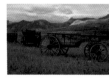

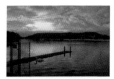

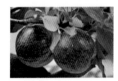

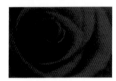

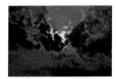

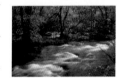

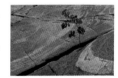

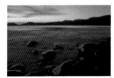

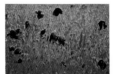

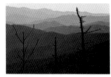

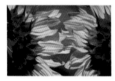

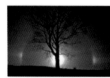

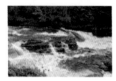

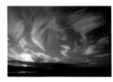

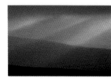

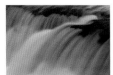

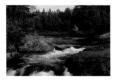

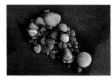

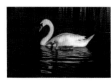

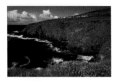

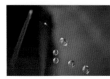

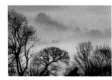

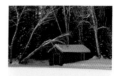

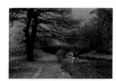

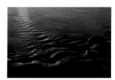

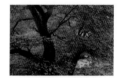

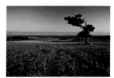

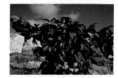

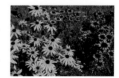

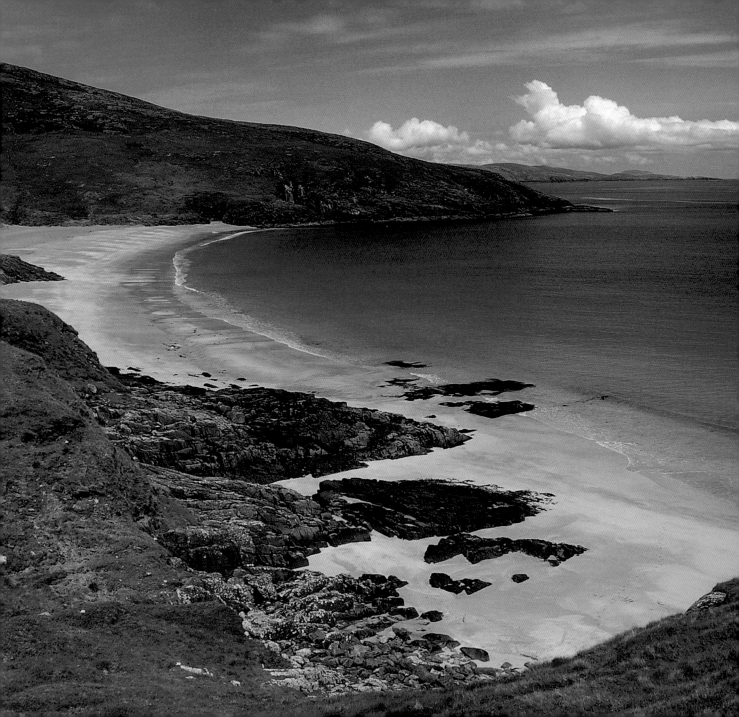

Part Three

My Pictures

Attach pictures, notes, and other items
with meaning for you.

Credits

Page 7: Clayoquat traditional poem from John Colombo Robert, *Songs of the Indians, Volume II.* (1983). Ottawa, ON: Oberon Press, p. 27.

Page 14: Hebrew Scripture from *The Judaica Press Complete Tanach.* (1969–1997). Translated by Rabbi A. J. Rosenberg. Yeshayahu 43:1b–2a. New York: Judaica Press.

Page 15: Julian of Norwich from *The Revelation of Divine Love in Sixteen Showings: Made to Dame Julian of Norwich.* (1994). Translated by M. L. del Mastro. Ligouri, MO: Ligouri Publications, p. 183.

Page 16: Christian Scripture from *The Holy Bible: New Revised Standard Version.* (1990). John 14:1–3a. Grand Rapids, MI: Zondervan Bible Publishers.

Page 17: Crowfoot quoted in Ethel Brant Monture, *Canadian Portraits: Brant, Crowfoot, Oronhyatekha, Famous Indians.* (1960). Toronto: Clarke, Irwin and Company, Ltd., p. 128.

Page 24: Anne Knight, personal friend with terminal cancer.

Page 27: Ascribed to Rossiter Worthington Raymond in Michael Counsell (Ed.), *Two Thousand Years of Prayer.* (2004). Norwich, UK: Canterbury Press, p. 424. All effort has been made to find the copyright owners of this quotation, without success.

Page 29: Rabbi Harold Kushner from *When Bad Things Happen to Good People.* (1981). New York: Avon Books, p. 134.

Page 30: Muslim Scripture from *The Holy Qur'an*, Fourteenth Edition. (1999). Translated by Abdullah Yusuf Ali. 11. Hud 56a. Elmhurst, NY: Tahrike Tarsile Qur'an.

Page 35: Rachel Naomi Remen from "Choose Life!" in *Kitchen Table Wisdom: Stories that Heal,* by Rachel Naomi Remen, M.D. (1996). Used by permission of Riverhead Books, an imprint of Penguin Books (USA), Inc., New York. Page 199.

Page 36–37: Hebrew Scriptures from *The Judaica Press Complete Tanach*, Tehillim 23:4 and 139:7–10.

Page 38: Christian Scripture from *The Holy Bible: New Revised Standard Version*, Romans 8:38 and 39.

Page 39: Rabindranath Tagore quoted in *Illustrations Unlimited*. (1988). Edited by J. S. Hewett. Wheaton, IL: Tyndale Publishers, p. 148. This is an out of print edition.

Page 40: Elisabeth Kübler-Ross from *Death: The Final Stage of Growth*, Reprinted with the permission of Simon & Schuster, Inc. Copyright © 1975 by Elisabeth Kübler-Ross. All rights reserved. Page 166.

Page 50: Miriam Greenspan from *Healing Through the Dark Emotions: The Wisdom of Grief, Fear, and Despair*. (2003). Boston: Shambala Publications, Inc., p. 100.

Page 51: Christian Scripture from *The Holy Bible: New Revised Standard Version*, Philippians 4:8.

Page 55: Arlene Cotter from *From This Moment On: A Guide for Those Recently Diagnosed with Cancer*. (1999). New York: Random House, pp. 404–405.

Acknowledgments

I MUST BEGIN BY paying tribute to my sister Dorothy, whose vibrant and valiant character inspired the love and motivation to assemble these materials in the first place. She is sorely missed.

It was Deborah Romeyn, a body work specialist who works extensively with people with cancer, who first encouraged me to attempt this larger project. Thank you, Deb.

Thanks are also owed to Monique Vandale, Heather Watson-Burgess, James Watson-Burgess, Susan Anderson, and Anne Knight, who sorted through the pages of material I eventually assembled and who helped me to narrow the options down into something manageable. After them, I owe deep gratitude to Tom Roche, Margaret Clarke, Patricia Frain, Fred Nelson, Patti Finlay, Jill Taylor-Brown, and Dr. Harvey Chochinov, each of whom is a care professional who reviewed an early version of this book and provided valuable feedback. I also owe thanks to Ranya Haskins for her input.

The people at Health Professions Press have been wonderful, especially Mary Magnus, Director of Publications, who saw the potential in this project early on and who guided me through the many hoops and hurdles of publication. Thank you, Mary.

Then there is Maggie Sale, whose artistic nature photographs illuminate the pages of this book. Maggie has been a brilliant collaborator—creative, thoughtful, and a delight to work with. Although this book is mine conceptually and in terms of text, I am certain there will be those who will be drawn to it again and again because of the exquisite photographs. I am very grateful to have had Maggie's skills and friendship throughout this process.

Finally, I must express my heartfelt love and appreciation to Moe, whose constancy and encouragement have seen me through this and many other interesting developments in our life together.

About the Author and Photographer

Linda Watson, M.R.E., M.Div., Th.M. As a former pastoral and supportive care professional, Linda Watson has been drawn again and again to work with the dying and the bereaved. With master's degrees in religious education, divinity, and theology from McMaster University in Hamilton, Ontario, and the University of Toronto, Ms. Watson has worked in parish ministry and served as the Peer Support and Supportive Care Coordinator of a breast cancer resource center in Winnipeg, Manitoba. Unafraid to engage with people who were nearing the end of life, Ms. Watson was often the one to move in close and become a trusted companion of people who were dying and their loved ones. Through her work, she learned some of the questions to ask, some of the silences to leave hanging, and some of the words to offer when it was time. Her counseling and theological training, plus her own life experiences, have combined to enable her to be a positive presence—at bedsides and elsewhere—for those facing death. Much of her accumulated wisdom and experience is collected in the words found in these pages in the hopes of helping those whose lives and deaths she cannot directly touch.

Maggie Sale. Originally from England, Maggie Sale has made her home in Canada since 1974. As a Toronto-based photographer, she has traveled widely and enjoys combining landscape and nature photography with her travels. Her images have been published in a number of magazines and books in Canada, the United States, and the United Kingdom. Ms. Sale's images have also appeared in a number of exhibitions.

Ms. Sale is a member of the Canadian Association for Photographic Art as well as the Etobicoke Camera Club in Toronto. She is a photographic Judge and Presenter with the Greater Toronto Council of Camera Clubs. You can see more of her images at: http://www. maggiesale.ca.